Leech Therapy in Traditional Medicine

(Hirudotherapy)

By

Syed I Hasan MD (PSM)
Md Tanwir Alam MD (PSM)
Rajiv Gandhi University, Bangalore
India

CS Independent Publishing Platform, South Carolina, North Charleston, USA

Book Details

Paperback: 135 pages
Publisher: CS Independent Publishing Platform; 2nd edition (December, 2015)
Language: English
ISBN-10: 1517784433
ISBN-13: 978-1517784430
Product Dimensions: 6 x 9 inches

Corresponding email: izhunaz@gmail.com

Contact: 91-8287833547

Leech Therapy in traditional medicine
First Edition: 2014, Second Ed 2015
Publisher: CS Independent Publishing Platform; 2nd edition

Notice

Knowledge and practice in medical field are constantly changing. As new research and experience broaden our knowledge simultaneously present treatment trends are becoming dangerous rather than solving the ailments due to their unavoidable side-effects, people are looking for alternative like leech therapy. Medical experts are advicing and luring towardas this basic and effective unani therapy (leech therapy).Changes in practice, treatment and leech procedures may become necessary or appropriate. Readers are advised to check the most current information provided on procedures adviced, administered/applied, verify the recommendation for therapy, the method and duration of application and contraindications. It is the responsibility of the practitioner, relying on their own experience and knowledge of the patient, to make diagnoses, to determine indications and the best treatment for each individual patient according to basic concepts of treatment and to take all appropriate safety precautions. To the fullest extent of the law, neither the Publisher nor the Author assumes any liability for any injury and/or damage to persons or property arising out or related to any use of the material or procedure contained in this book.

Syed I Hasan
Md Tanwir Alam

About the book

Blood letting is an ancient medical procedure comprises of leeching, wet cupping and Venesection; still in use across the world. The evidence of use of leeches for blood letting procedure can be traced back in ancient system of medicine like Greco-roman, Indian and Arabic medicine. In early of 19th century their uses were very common among European surgeons for the means of natural and cosmetic healing in superficial and other surgical cut. Now a days leeching is an established therapeutic modality among Indian system of medicine (*Unani* and Ayurveda). It is being used for various diseases like varicosity, varicose and other non healing ulcers, warts, Melasma (Chloasma), hypertension, local congestion and joints pain etc. Inspite of that, standard operative procedure (SOPs) for leeching is yet to develop. In this book author comprises the possible indications of leech therapy along with procedures, safety concerns, historical perspective, surgical operative standards, and contraindication of the same described in *traditional* system of medicine.

This book is doctor-friendly because it would help the alternative medical practitioners involved in providing not only curative services, but also preventive and promotive services to the community at large, motivating them to a healthier, and happier life.

Despite our sincere efforts to make the book accurate and comprehensive as we could, it is possible there may be some gaps or errors in the book. We would be most grateful to the readers, if these deficiencies are pointed out so that can be removed in the next edition. We also invite healthy suggestions from all readers to help us improve the quality of book and achieve the purpose with which it has been written. All such feedback would be carefully considered and gratefully acknowledged.

Syed I Hasan

Md Tanwir Alam

"If we all treat each other like we treat ourselves what a wonderful place earth would be"

INDEX

INTRODUCTION

Throughout human history, a well documented natural medical aid has come from medical leeches. Hirudo medicinalis is the most common species of leech used in the medical arena, but other species are used depending on your location on the globe.

Medicinal leeches have had a place in the doctor's medical kit for centuries because they have proven themselves often to be the most effective treatment. Leeches were especially useful treating wounds and saving lives on the European battlefield in the 18th and 19th centuries. Leech therapy is also is referenced in the Talmud and in Islamic and Unani texts. Today, they even have FDA approval as a medical device. Tens of thousands of medicinal leeches are supplied from specialty biofarms every year to hospitals in dozens of countries for reconstructive surgeries and skin grafts. The creatures' saliva is known to contain at least 15 enzymes with proven healing properties. The enzyme hirudin, for example, has a therapeutic effect on dangerous blood clots.

Hirudotherapy – the formal name for leech therapy – is making a comeback in the United States as an increasing number of people are looking for drug-free solutions for their health conditions. Leech therapy has been used to successfully treat thrombosis, cramped veins, heart disease, tinnitus, bruises, rheumatism, hemorrhoids, muscle complications, and numerous other conditions.

The therapeutic activity of the leech is not based on a single mechanism of action, but on a combination of multiple effects. The leech's saliva is truly extraordinary containing a number of chemical compounds useful in medicine. These include a local anesthetic that the leech uses to avoid detection by the host, the anti-coagulant hirudin that can help prevent heart attacks and strokes, a vasodilator and a prostaglandin that help reduce swelling. The leech's gut harbors a bacterium known as Aeromonan hydrophila. This bacterium aids in the digestion of ingested blood and produces an antibiotic that kills other bacteria that may cause putrefaction. The medical term for such a cornucopia of effects is called a "multifactorial mechanism."

The positive effect of hirudotherapy on the blood makes it very effective against difficult diseases such as hypertension, coronary heart disease, and atherosclerosis.

Leech therapy should always be administered by a trained professional. To achieve the greatest effect, it is necessary to have a well-developed understanding of the human body and particularly the circulatory system.

The therapy is relatively simple, inexpensive, and indispensable when it comes to many chronic diseases and performs as good as, if not better than, some conventional medical procedures which may be more costly, have higher risks of complications, and are usually accompanied by synthetic pharmaceutical drugs that can have nasty side effects.

In the case of a severe illness, the effects of leech therapy are felt almost immediately. The patient experiences reduced pain, diminished swelling, and a drop in body temperature. Moreover, leech therapy can be used to reduce the duration of a disease, prevent possible complications, and support a good state of health.

Leech therapy is not just a surface treatment. It is a complex process that should be regarded as a holistic treatment for the entire body, rather than a mechanical bleeding in one spot that benefits only a local issue.

Leeches have been used in medicine for thousands of years. Leeches remove blood ("phlebotomize") from their host, and they release pain-killing (anesthetic) and blood-thining (anticoaggulant) substances with their saliva. Live leeches are currently used to treat blood-congested limbs, which otherwise might die or require amputation, if the pooling blood cannot be removed any other way. They are also sometimes used to provide pain relief, and for many other therapeutic effects.

HISTORY OF LEECH THERAPY

The use of medicinal leeches is as old as the Pyramids. Literally, Records indicate that Egyptians used leech therapy more than 3,500 years ago and leeches (often mistakenly credited as cobras) are included in the hieroglyphics painted on the walls. The tombs of Egyptian pharaohs contained pictures of leeches, and descriptions of leech medical treatments appear in ancient Greek and Roman texts. The popularity of the use of leeches in the 18th and 19th century in Europe caused them to become scarce. Leech therapy was used to treat a wide range of conditions.

Herophilos (335-280 BC) was a Greek physician who was the first scientist to systematically perform scientific dissections of human cadavers and is deemed to be the first anatomist. Hippocrates (460BC-370BC), another Greek physician, is referred to as the "father of medicine." He was the first physician to reject superstitions, legends, and beliefs that credited supernatural or divine forces causing illness.

Both physicians used medicinal leeches, amongst other methods, to remove blood from a patient to "balance the humours." The four humours of ancient medical philosophy were blood, phlegm, black bile, and yellow bile. The belief at the time was that these four humours must be kept in balance in order for the human body to function properly. Any disease or illness was thought to be a result of an imbalance of these humours. The dominant humour was believed to be blood.

However, it was Aelius Galenus (AD 129 – 200), a prominent physician and philosopher and the most accomplished medical researcher of the Roman era, who introduced blood letting to Rome. His theories dominated and influenced Western medical science for well over a millennium. Of the four humours, Galen believed that blood was the dominant humour and the one in most need of control. Romans were the first to use the HIRUDO name for leeches.

Leech therapy, or hirudotherapy, survived the fall of the Roman Empire and remained popular throughout the Middle Ages. Over the centuries it remained an integral part of treating disease and illnesses all around the world. Bloodletting in its various forms was especially popular in the young United States of America. Dr. Benjamin Rush, a signatory of the Declaration of Independence, saw the state of the arteries as the key to disease, recommending higher than ever levels of bloodletting.

Sometimes, "bloodletting" was overdone; it worked so well in so many cases, some tried to use it for everything. At the beginning of the 1800s French physician Poliniere asked, "Leeches – immense good, or terrible scourge?"

Dr. Henry Clutterbuck, lecturing at the Royal College of Physicians, stated in 1840, "blood-letting is a remedy which, when judiciously employed, is hardly possible to estimate too highly."

Indeed, by the mid 1800s the demand for leeches was so high that the French imported about forty million leeches a year for medical purposes, and in the next decade, England imported six million leeches a year from France alone, since the leech production from their own farm near Oxford were insufficient. And it wasn't just Europe – there was an explosion in the use of leeches in Asia and the Middle East.

Bloodletting was recommended by Sir William Osler in the 1923 edition of his textbook The Principles and Practice of Medicine.

With the advent of antibiotics in the mid 20th century, leeches fell out of favor. But not for long, in the second half of the 20th century leeches made a comeback with the advent of microsurgery such as plastic and reconstructive surgeries. In operations such as these, one of the biggest problems that arise is venous congestion due to inefficient venous drainage. This condition is known as venous insufficiency. If this congestion is not cleared up quickly, the blood will clot and arteries that bring the tissues their necessary nourishment will become plugged and the tissues will die. It is here where the leeches come in handy. After being applied to the required site, they suck the excess blood, reducing the swelling in the tissues and promoting healing by allowing fresh, oxygenated blood to reach the area until normal circulation can be restored. The leeches also secrete an anticoagulant (known as hirudin) that prevents the clotting of the blood.

In June, 2004, the Food and Drug administration (FDA) gave approval for the commercial marketing of Medicinal Leeches and determined that leeches are medical devices because they meet the definition of a medical device.

Medical research and the use of leeches never stopped in some parts of the world, especially in Germany and Russia. So it is little wonder that both countries achieved the highest level in overall research on medicinal leeches and Russia became the biggest producer of Hirudo Medicinalis in the world.

The popularity of leech therapy began centuries ago when there was little research or scientific facts available to back up the benefits – people just knew it worked. Today, however, we do have proven facts and studies of the numerous advantages of using leech therapy.

Today leeches are on the cusp of not only enjoying a revival for known health benefits, but there are constant new discoveries based on thorough medical research about positive effects of the substances medicinal leeches introduce into the human body (and animals as well!) during the hirudotherapy treatments.

Leech therapy has a long history. Records indicate that Egyptians used leech therapy 3,500 years ago. Leech treatments were very popular during the Middle Ages. Again leech therapy became was commonly practiced in the 1800's by American physicians treating a variety of diseases.

In the 1980, medicinal leech therapy got a big boost by plastic surgeons who used leeches to relieve venous congenstion, especially in transplant surgery. This use of leech therapy ("hirudotherapy") provides a good example of its current status. When appendages are re-attached following traumatic amputation, it is often possible to reconnect the largfer arterial blood vessels, but not the thinner, more delicate venous vessels. The body will eventually develop the necessary venous connections to drain the area of oxygen-depleted blood; but if this does not occur rapidly enough, the pooling venous blood can produce enough swelling and pressure that fresh arterial blood may no longer be able to enter the re-connected limb. In this situation, leeches are used to drain the local blood and decompress the pressure within the grafted limb, otherwise at risk of necrosis (death).

Today, Medicinal leeches are also used in the treatment of other veinous deseases such as thrombophlebitis, as well as angina pectoris, arthritis, hematomas, and even tinnitus.

Leech therapy's back in India

A few years ago when Hollywood actress Demi Moore said she let leeches suck her blood as part of a therapy to look fresh and young it made headlines. This ancient medical therapy of using leeches for clinical bloodletting to treat certain health conditions is making a comeback of sorts in India where the therapy is said to have originated.

Leeches (or Hirudo Medicinalis) are segmented worms from the Annelida family with suckers at the ends of their body. A leech can consume between 5 and 15 ml of blood- or four-six times their body weight in a single feed. The bite of a leech is not painful as it releases an anaesthetic to prevent the hosts from feeling them.

Many people are now taking to leech therapy to treat conditions ranging from blood pressure to gout, from healing wounds to even hair fall. Only the medicinal leeches are used for treatment, which are brown, red striped and olive-coloured.

LEECH THERAPY IN UNANI: HISTORICAL PERSPECTIVE

In *Unani*, Arabic word *"Alaq"* is used for leech. *"Irasale alaq"* means application of leeches and word *"Taleeq"* is used in equivalent to leech therapy. In short we can say *"Taleeq"* or *"Irsale Alaq"* means, "leeching". The word *"Alaq"* is the plural of *"alqa"*, which means, "leech". Leech therapy was first introduced by Hippocrates a famous *Unani* physician and father of medicine. Furthermore Galen classified Leech therapy as a method of treatment and prevention of health. Famous *Unani* physicians like: Rofus, Arkaghanees, Razi, Majoosi, Maseehi, Zahravi, Ibn Sina, Ibn Hubal Badhdadi, Ismail Jurjani, Akbar Arzani And Abdul Hameed Bhopali etc. have recommended *Irasale Alaq* in their writings for various ailments. There was boom in Leech therapy during middle ages. After a long gap the leech therapy was brought back into the medical domain in the middle of 20th century.

NATURAL HISTORY OF LEECHES

The medicinal leech (Hirudo medicinalis) is a segmented worm (Phylum: Annelida). This phylum includes the Polychaetes, the Oligochaetes (earthworms) and the Hirudinea (leeches).

Leeches have two "suckers," one at each end. The caudal (back end) suction cup helps the leech to ambulate on dry surfaces, and to attach to its host; the rostral (front end) suction cup also contains the mouth with three sharp jaws that leave a Y-shaped bite.

The medicinal leech lives in clean waters. Leeches swim free in the water, with an undulating motion. When attached to its host for feeding, the leech remains in place for 30 minutes to 6 hours or more, as it fills with blood. During feeding, H. medicinalis can suck 5 - 15 mL of blood --- several times its own body weight.

Leech saliva contains several bioactive substances, including anti-cooaggulants, vaso-dilators, and anesthetics. Hirudin, a potent anticoagulant in leech saliva, inhibits the conversion of fibrinogen to fibrin, preventing blood from clotting. Indeed, a wound may continue to bleed for many hours after the leech has already detached.

The benefits of leech therapy are due, in large part, to the anti-coaggulant effects, vasodilatory effects, and anesthetic effects of these biochemicals, as well as the physical effects of blood letting (phlebotomy).

Like a snake, the leech periodically must shed its skin. The leech is hermaphtroditic, having both male and female elements. Fertilization and egg-laying usually occur during the spring, summer, and winter months. Young leeches feed on the blood of small water animals (frogs, toads or fish). Leeches may not be ready for medical application until they are several years old.

DEFINITION OF HIRUDOTHERAPY

A simple healing principle lies at the heart of all hirudo-miracles. Hirudin is the naturally occurring peptide of the Hirudo medicinalis (medicinal leech). This is a four-inch long carnivorous, hermaphroditic segmented worm. It has a sucker on each end, five pairs of eyes, and 32 nerve bundles (or brains) in the middle. This buccal secretion from the salivary glands is best known for its anticoagulant property. This is fundamental for the alimentary habit of hematophagy since it keeps the blood flowing through the leech after the initial phlebotomy on the host's skin. During the feeding process, leeches secrete a complete mixture of pharmacologically active substances, with hirudin being the best-known component of the saliva.

It is difficult to extract large amounts of hirudin from the natural sources, however in June 2004, the FDA lent its seal of approval on the centuries old medical device of leeches. The traditional medical use of leeches is for skin grafts on burn patients and reattachment surgery; and the natural medical uses are more far reaching.

While there are roughly 600 leech species only about 15 are classified as "medicinal leeches." Today, the medicinal leeches are farmed in pristine conditions, shipped and stored for a one-time use as they are disposed of after the treatment. There is no risk of indirect transfer of infectious diseases from one patient to another, nor has the transmission of other pathogens (bacterial or viral) within this context of leech therapy been observed.

While they are raised in sterile conditions, Aeromonas hydrophila, a bacterium that prevents putrefaction of the leech's blood meal and supplies enzymes crucial to its digestion, 20% of patients can become infected by this bacterium, especially those with weakened immune systems. Aeromonas also kills other bacteria; and for some reason, staph cannot grow inside a leech. Perhaps it is the inhospitable condition within the leech or something the Aeromonas produces that inhibits the growth of staph.

The action of the hirudin is the ability to inhibit the procoagulant activity of thrombin. In fact, hirudin is the most potent natural inhibitor of thrombin as it dissolves the formation of clots and thrombi; thus having a therapeutic value in blood coagulation disorders, superficial varicose veins, and skin hematomas. An advantage over commonly used prescription anticoagulants is that hirudin does not interfere with the biological activity of other serum proteins and can act on complexed thrombin.

However, the salivary glands contain more than 100 bioactive substances with more benefits than anticoagulation. These include: anti-edematous, analgesic, bacteriostatic, eliminates microcirculation disorders, detoxifies the organism thereby reducing complications such as infarct or stroke, restores damaged vascular permeability (organs and tissues), reduces blood pressure, increases immune system activity and eliminates oxygen starvation.

LEECH TAXONOMY AND MORPHOLOGY

Leeches (Euhirudinea) were first named by Linnaeus in 1758 AD. They are related to the phylum Annelida, class Clitellata. In general, early studies classified leeches into 4 subclasses, 3 orders, 10 families, 16 subfamilies, 131 genera and more than 696 species. Recently, taxonomists identified more than 1000 leech species. Leech size varies among families and can reach up to 20 cm in length, in addition to some giant species, such as the Amazonian leech, Haementaria ghilianii, which is about 50 cm in length. A classic leech body consists of many segments divided as two preoral, nonmetameric segments, and 32 postoral metameres (somites). Somites are subdivided into 2-16 external annuli, and the annulation pattern can be considered as a diagnostic feature for leech genus and species. Sensory structures, such as eyes, oculiform spots, papillae and sensilla are also used by taxonomists to identify genus, and species. Typically, a leech has anterior and posterior suckers. Some leeches related to the order Rhynchobdellida have a large anterior sucker with a small jaw-less mouth and protrusible muscular proboscis. Others from the order Arhynchobdellida possess a simple anterior sucker with a wide mouth, which may or may not have jaws such as in hirudinids and erpobdellids, respectively. Suckers are very essential during movement (inchworm-like locomotion) and for attachment to host surface. Leeches breathe through the skin and they are considered as hermaphrodites, but always require another leech for fertilization.

THE BIOLOGY OF LEECH FEEDING

Based on feeding habits, leeches are divided into two major groups. The first group includes the predacious leeches, which are predators of many invertebrates. The second group, named the sanguivorous leeches are ectoparasites that feed on the blood of vertebrates including human. With the help of suckers and the biting jaws, leeches are able to absorb prey blood]. It is interesting to note that leeches generally suck 2-20 ml of blood within 10-30 min, then drop-off spontaneously after being completely engorged with no immediate desire of more feeding.

Leeches, both sanguivorous and predacious, digest their food in their intestine. The sanguivorous species only store blood inside their body for months. Actually, the digestion process of blood in hematophagous leeches undergoes many slow stages allowing leeches to store the ingested blood for up to 18 months. Symbiotic bacteria named Aeromonas spp., located in the leech's gut, secrete enzymes that help not only in breaking down the components of the ingested blood, but also in producing antibiotics to prevent blood putrefaction after a long storage period in leech crop. Furthermore, another presumed role of these enzymes is to prevent B complex deficiency, which often occurs in blood nutrition-depending animals.

AIMS OF LEECHING

- The main aim of Leeching is to clean the morbid matter from the site of the disease.

- To absorb sanguineous matters more efficiently from deeper tissues as compared to *Hijamah* (wet cupping) and *fasd* (Venesection) with little or no pain.

- Leeching is the counter part of Venesection in children
- To do *Imala* (diversion of morbid matter)
- To relieve the pain.
- To relieve venous congestion, more effectively than conventional therapies

CLINICAL PRACTICE OF LEECH THERAPY

The application of leech therapy is simple: leeches are gently placed in the area needed, and allowed to attach and engorge for the next 6-12 hours, after which they will release. The entire course of treatment may require one to 6 treatments or more, depending upon the goals and rate of response.

Leeches (Hirudo Medicinalis) have been used medically for more than 1500 years. Originally used to remove "bad blood," the leech is now used extensively by reconstructive surgeons needing to remove stagnant blood from a flap or reattached limb. When the venous blood does not return to the heart, it pools in the wounded area, increasing pressure and preventing fresh arterial blood from entering the area with oxygen and nutrients. The venous blood must be removed and the pressure must be reduced in order to save the flap or limb. The leech is able to do this exceptionally well, because its saliva contains important biochemicals, including vasodilators, anticoagulants, and anesthetics.

The leech will withdraw approximately 5 ml (one teaspoon) of blood. Further therapeutic benefit of leech therapy comes after the leech is removed, during which up to 50 mls of blood will continue to ooze, for up to 48 hours. More leeches attached to the site mean more blood will be removed. After 3-7 days, the veins have usually reconnected themselves such that the blood is no longer pooling in the limb. Normal color and pressure should return to the area, as arterial blood circulates easily in the damaged zone. By that time, the wound will be able to heal, without further phlebotomy (leech therapy).

The application of leeches to the patient is relatively simple, but does require care. As few as one, or as many as 6 or more leeches may be required for a wound, depending upon its size and its clinical response. The greatest number of leeches should be applied to the area of maximal venous congestion.

The patient's skin must be cleaned thoroughly with soap and water, and then rinsed with distilled, non-chlorinated water. A gauze barrier around the area intended for the leech will help prevent the leech from wandering away from the site where it's attachment is desired. It can be carried to the site by hand, or it can be placed within a 5 cc plastic syringe (plunger removed) and then applied to the wound site, containing the leech until it is attached.

If the leech is reluctant to bite, it might be necessary to entice it with a tiny droplet of blood, drawn from the wound site with a needle prick.

Once the leech is attached, it will likely remain safely in place until fully distended. The gauze square can be removed and used elsewhere without disturbing the animal;however, it is important that the site be checked continuously to insure that the leech hasn't moved. The leech will let go of the patient (host) when it is finished (usually within an hour).

LEECH THERAPY FOR ARTHRITIS

Leech therapy is considered by those with experience with it to be the best therapeutic treatment for arthritis. The saliva of leeches introduces an anti-inflammatory agent to the joint, and the saliva also acts as a pain reliever due to the anesthetic component. Also, the saliva of leeches acts as a histamine and a vasodilator, which benefit the arthritis sufferer..

Leech therapy, also known as hirudotherapy, remains the best hope for treating arthritis pain, far surpassing any prescription drug on the market. Given the benefits of the saliva of leeches, patients have reported a surge in energy, as well as the end of their arthritis pain. Patients have also reported a better night's sleep after having leech therapy.

Arthritis treatment with leeches is often a one time treatment. The treatment usually takes only an hour, with a small leech positioned on the point of the arthritis pain. Because of the natural anesthetic released by the leech, there is no discomfort or pain with the procedure. Leeches also act to filter infection from the blood which also aids in inflammation and pain relief. Once the procedure is over, most patients report better movement and comfort by the day after the treatment. In most cases, treatment doesn't require repeating for up to six months.

There are no side effects, and information on leech therapy shows pain relief for nearly a year.

LEECH THERAPY FOR CARDIOVASCULAR DISEASES

Cardiovascular disease has long been a main indication for leech therapy. The prominent doctor Nickolay I. Pirogov of Russia was among the first in modern history to treat heart disease with leeches in the 1800s. Good results have been seen even in cases of sclerotic changes in blood vessel walls.

Atherosclerosis is when the blood vessel walls become thicker and harder due to "thick" and sticky blood. The artery walls – particularly at the "Y" junctions around the heart, neck, and large arteries of the legs – are scarred as a result of the turbulent process of thick and sticky blood moving through them. Then Nature lays down cholesterol as a repair mechanism and the arteries narrow. This is a chronic vascular disease.

Cholesterol is not the cause of heart disease; it is a symptom. If the artery walls were not "nicked" by the blood moving through them, cholesterol would not be called upon.

Blood actually thickens as it slows down – think of a blood clot as an extreme case. When the heart fills with blood after contraction, slower-moving red blood cells cling together more easily. This makes the blood more viscous – more thick and sticky. When the heart squeezes to make the next contraction, the blood flows faster and becomes less viscous. So blood viscosity fluctuates with each heartbeat. Blood viscosity determines how hard our heart has to work, and how much injury "thick" and therefore abrasive blood cells can inflect on artery walls. Cholesterol is merely the body's response to protect injuries areas from further abrasion.

Having more viscous blood can be likened to the phrase, "death by 1000 cuts." Blood gets thick as a result of the modern lifestyle and diet factors which are driving up rates of chronic disease. For example, high triglycerides increase viscosity. Triglycerides – a measure of fats in the bloodstream – respond quickly to a meal, particularly one with a lot of fat, sugar, or alcohol. (When we eat, calories are released. Excess calories are converted into triglycerides which are stored in the fat cells and used to supply energy when required. High levels of triglycerides are directly linked with dietary imbalances in most of the cases.) An elevated triglyceride level is a strong risk factor for heart attack among middle-aged and elderly men, a stronger risk factor than total cholesterol alone.

The Edinburgh Artery Study of the 1990s observed 4860 men for five years and found that 20 percent of men with highest viscosity had 55 percent of the major cardiovascular events. Only 4 percent of those with low viscosity had any significant cardiovascular event.

It is well established that pre-menopausal women have fewer cardiovascular events. The monthly blood loss has a very significant effect on blood viscosity because her blood contains perhaps 80 percent more new, young blood cells. Younger red blood cells are less likely to clump together.

With this brief understanding of the hazards of viscous blood, you can begin to see why leech therapy has long been a strong defense against heart disease.

The hirudin in the leech saliva opposes the process of blood clotting. Hirudin is a polypeptide, which has highly potent antiprotease activity with a strict specificity for thrombin, meaning it is able to inactivate fibrin-bound thrombin. Other factors can also stabilize the blood clotting system, produce a beneficial effect on the vascular wall, and improve microcirculation which leads to improved blood circulation and oxygen supply of all internal organs. The enzymes leeches deposit with their saliva prevent blood from becoming thick, thereby promoting better blood circulation not only in the heart but to other parts of the body.

Leeches prompt some blood loss and thus prompt the body to make new blood cells which are more flexible than older blood cells.

There are about 90 miles of veins in the body, and hirudotherapy can clean them and make them stronger and more flexible.

Hypertension – high blood pressure – is a measurement of the force against the walls of your arteries as your heart pumps blood through your body. You are more likely to be told your blood pressure is too high as you get older. This is because your blood vessels become stiffer as you age. When that happens, your blood pressure goes up. High blood pressure increases your chance of having a stroke, heart attack, heart failure, kidney disease, and early death.

In the treatment of hypertension with leeches, the effect is twofold. First, there is a decrease in the volume of blood circulating in the bloodstream and that directly lessens the pressure along blood vessel walls.

Second, the bio-active agents in the saliva exert significant hypotensive (pressure reducing) effects.

With hirudotherapy, it is often possible to reduce the dose of prescription drugs, and sometimes end their use.

For treating hypertension, the leeches are generally placed on body parts like upper back, neck, and chest.

Varicose veins are unattractive, but the disease can give rise to the dangerously threatening complication of thrombophlebitis. Surgery is a common treatment, but often the varicose veins return. People have become to understand the value of hirudotherapy as a very effective treatment.

Hirudotherapy does not preclude other treatments, but the use of leeches for varicose veins dramatically reduces the need for surgery, post surgical complications, and the downtime of recovery.

LEECH THERAPY FOR ALOPECIA

Baldness or alopecia is a very common condition where an individual loses hair. Hair loss can occur in various parts of the body, but the most common area is the scalp. Men are generally affected more but women can also suffer from this condition, often causing embarrassment.

Individuals who have parents suffering from this condition will likely develop alopecia in the future. It has also been suggested that autoimmune diseases can cause alopecia, where hair follicles are being attacked by the body, causing suppression of growth. The body sends signals for T-cell lymphocytes to attach themselves to hair follicles, causing inflammation on the site and thereby suppressing hair growth.

Another very common cause of alopecia is a fungal infection of the scalp or dandruff, resulting in weakened hair follicles and subsequent hair loss. It has also been found that stress can cause some people to develop hair loss or alopecia.

Leech therapy is known to increase blood circulation, therefore when therapy is applied to thinning or bald areas, the increase of blood circulation helps enhance the concentration and delivery of nutrients that assist in making hair follicles strong, thereby assisting in the promotion of hair growth.

People suffering alopecia caused by fungal infections or dandruff can also benefit through the antibacterial component in the leeches saliva, which helps combat fungal infections.

LEECH THERAPY FOR INFANTILE CEREBRAL PALSY

Our brains, although enclosed in a very thick skull, is still a very fragile organ. It can be damaged very easily even if we are still in the womb, such as in the case of infantile cerebral palsy. Since our brain controls all of the functions of our body, a person suffering from this kind of brain disorder is left with motor and sensory impairments.

Infantile cerebral palsy is an injury of the brain. It can happen during the fetal development of the child, during the birth of the child or during the first three years of the child's life. This brain injury can result in one-sided involvement or total involvement of the body. Muscle tightness, weakness or involuntary muscle movements can also be seen in patients with infantile cerebral palsy.

Because the brain is damaged, mental retardation and physical growth problems are present as well as vision and hearing problems. Also, there are behavioral as well as social impairments.

A lot of things or factors can cause infantile cerebral palsy. During fetal development, the fetus may suffer from temporary loss of blood supply, resulting in brain damage. Likewise, when the brain is deprived of blood and oxygen during the child birthing process, the result may also be infantile cerebral palsy. The developing brain can also be damaged by an infection acquired by the mother while the fetus is still in the womb, such as in the case of rubella virus infection. Drugs and alcohol intake during pregnancy also increases the risk of the child developing infantile cerebral palsy.

Other causes of this brain disorder are severe head trauma leading to hemorrhage and subsequent damage to the brain. Diseases and illnesses contracted during the first three years of a child's life may also lead to this brain disorder; an example of such illnesses is meningitis.

One of the unpleasant side effects of medications used in patients with infantile cerebral palsy is vascular complications where an individual can suffer swelling and bleeding. Vascular complications compromise health, which can lead to more difficulties. Swelling can also reduce blood flow to the brain and although the brain disorder is not progressive, further injury can result from complications, which may cause possible degeneration of healthy brain cells.

Using medications in conjunction with leech therapy can greatly reduce the risk of vascular complications.

There are many enzymes in leech saliva that are very beneficial to the human body.

Anticoagulation enzymes are known to help blood flow freely to the brain, preventing thickening, which can lead to blood clots. If there are blood clots already present in the body, enzymes from the leech's saliva will help dissolve them so blood can flow freely.

Another enzyme in the leech's saliva is a histamine-like enzyme, which helps dilate the vessels, promoting good blood flow to the brain. Swelling in the brain is also reduced by anti-inflammatory agents, which are again found in the leech's saliva.

Antibacterial agents in the saliva of the leech can eliminate harmful bacteria, therefore boosting the immune system and helping it ward off further infection.

LEECH THERAPY FOR HEPATITIS

Signs and symptoms of hepatitis vary, depending upon the cause of liver inflammation. Some people experience flu-like symptoms, vomiting, nauseous or loss of appetite and diarrhea. General body weakness can be felt, as well as muscle aches or tenderness on the right side of the body underneath the ribcage. People suffering long-term hepatitis can have a distinct yellowing of the skin and eyes; in fact, there are many signs and symptoms, depending upon the kind of hepatitis.

There are many things that can cause hepatitis, but viruses are the most common. Viruses can be transmitted when an individual ingests contaminated food or water, undergoes an exchange of blood or when individuals have unprotected sex with an infected partner. Drug addicts who share needles with other addicts are also susceptible to hepatitis.

Aside from viruses that can cause hepatitis, alcoholics can also develop alcoholic hepatitis, where the liver becomes inflamed due to the excessive amount of consumed alcohol. Alcoholic hepatitis can lead to cirrhosis of the liver caused by long-term alcohol consumption.

There are also a number of medications and drugs that can damage the liver when used over a long period of time, for example some antihypertensive drugs, antibiotics and antidepressants can cause some inflammation to the liver.

Leech therapy has been used in the treatment of many illnesses for thousands of years.

A healthy blood supply is needed to fight off infection and inflammation in the liver and beneficial enzymes found in the saliva of leeches include anti-inflammatory enzymes which help reduce swelling as well as histamine-like enzymes that act to vasodilate the blood vessels, further enhancing blood flow. There are also antibacterial components in leech saliva that help fight disease.

LEECH THERAPY FOR ENDOMETRIOSIS

It has been found that leech therapy is very beneficial to women who are suffering from Endometriosis.

The cause of pain in Endometriosis is brought about by clots of blood clinging to the uterine wall as well as swelling of the area, further trapping toxins that can greatly increase pain.

The saliva in leeches is rich with enzymes that can prevent coagulation of blood which leads to blood clots. Once these enzymes have dissolved the blood clots and restored a normal flow of blood into the uterus, toxins are flushed away.

Another important compound in leech's saliva is the anti-inflammatory enzymes, which aid in the reduction of inflammation. Once inflammation subsides, blood can flow freely into vessels, which are further dilated by the vasodilator agents in leech's saliva.

There are also antibacterial agents in the leech's saliva, which further protect the uterus and surrounding areas from bacterial infection, which can also cause pain and swelling.

LEECH THERAPY FOR DENTAL ISSUES

Back in the days of cowboys and the American West, when a tooth got inflamed, people pulled it out – often with pliers. The source of irritation was gone, the abscess drained, and the mouth healed.

But modern dentists will perform a "root canal" – removal of the tooth's pulp which contains nerve fibers, arteries, veins, lymph vessels, and connective tissue. The dead tooth is left in the mouth. The emptied root cavity is filled, but over time, root canals leak and can be a source of constant "toxic drip" that feeds chronic diseases.

That infectious mechanism was documented a century ago by Dr. Weston A. Price, chairman of the Research Section of the American Dental Association (ADA) from 1914-1923. Dr. Price observed that when teeth which had been given a root canal treatment were removed from patients with kidney or heart disease, the patients almost always got better. He documented that when a removed root canal tooth was inserted under the skin of a rabbit, the rabbit would die within two days; when normal teeth were inserted, there was no adverse health effect and the rabbit survived. History tells us the ADA, however, wanted to promote root canals as a new service and turned a deaf ear to Dr. Price's research.

Hirudotherapy – the formal name for leech therapy – can often spare you the unfortunate legacy of a root canal.

A tooth's nerve and pulp can become irritated, inflamed, and infected due to deep decay, repeated dental procedures on a tooth such as fillings and crowns, a crack or chip in the tooth, or trauma to the face. When a tooth becomes infected, an abscess often forms. And that is your warning bell – with the abscess, comes pain. Your body is trying to get your attention because it needs help.

Leeches can be applied to the site of the abscess where they will drain the inflammation.

Anticoagulation agents increase blood flow in the gums, helping to eliminate toxins and allow delivery of nutrients to the affected area. These anti-coagulation agents also dissolve the blood clots that could be developed in the gums. The saliva in leech also contains antibacterial components that assist in reducing bacterial growth.

Using hirudotherapy instead of a root canal procedure provides an invaluable service. In the short-term, you are spared an expensive procedure in the dentist's office with needles of Novocain and a round of pharmaceutical antibiotics. In the long term, you will have saved a tooth and spared yourself the inadvertent creation of a toxic drip site.

The anti-inflammatory, immunostimulant, and analgesic effects of hirudotherapy have been used to treat various inflammatory processes in the oral cavity including periodontitis (chronic inflammatory process affecting the tissues surrounding the tooth), gingivitis (inflammation of the gums, abscess), and inflammation of the periosteum (covering of the tooth's bony socket).

LEECH THERAPY FOR DIGESTIVE SYSTEM DISEASES

Gastrointestinal diseases have become very common and almost all of them are chronic and accompanied by dysbiosis (gut dysfunction).

Medical leeches are effective on the root cause of so much gut dysfunction – inflammation. Leech saliva provides anti-inflammatory, analgesic, antibiotic, and normalizing metabolism effects. Leeches also have a positive effect on the overall condition of the nervous system.

LEECH THERAPY FOR DRUG, ALCOHOL DETOX

Prescription drugs can be just as addictive as illegal drugs. For example, hydrocodone, a prescription opiate, is synthetic heroin. It's indistinguishable from any other heroine as far as your brain and body is concerned.

Fleetwood Mac star Stevie Nicks said the biggest mistake she ever made was giving in to her friends and going to see a psychiatrist. He prescribed the anti-anxiety drug Klonopin, and, according to Nicks, the next eight years of her life were destroyed.

Today, prescription drugs cause more deaths and premature deaths than illegal drugs.

The body's reaction to the removal of a substance it has become dependent upon is called withdrawal. Withdrawal causes craving for more of the substance being removed. The period of time when the body is trying to overcome its addiction is called detoxification (detox).

Every time a person uses addictive drugs, residual amounts are stored in the body's fatty tissues. When the body metabolizes that tissue, the stored toxins are released into the bloodstream, stimulating the craving to use drugs and alcohol again. A holistic detoxification program removes the drug and alcohol residue stored in body tissues to put an end to the cravings.

Leeches have a unique ability to tunnel into the blood and lymph system and detoxify.

Our bodies hold about 5 quarts of blood that travel through some 60,000 miles of blood vessels. Impurities and pollutants in the blood find their way into all blood cells, tissues and organs of the body as the blood circulates.

Our bodies hold about 1 ½ quarts of lymph fluid. The lymphatic system is often called the body's garbage can because it carries away the waste that the cells cast off – cancer cells, nitrogenous wastes, trapped protein, fatty globules, pathogenic bacteria, infectious viruses, foreign substances, heavy metals, and other assorted matter.

Medicinal leeches act as a disposable syringe, tunneling into both the blood and the lymph systems. This prompts the body to release stored residues. Typically, what a person discharges over the next 12-36 hours is 30 percent blood, and 70 percent toxins.

Typically, people using hirudotherapy for drug or alcohol detox will tell us they know it is powerfully effective because the fluid they discharged after the first, and sometimes again after the second session, left no doubt that the leeches had accessed stored toxins more quickly than other methods they had tried.

As the residues decrease, the cravings decrease.

LEECH THERAPY FOR EYE DISEASES

Ever wondered how our ancestors dealt with their medical problems? Many very important medical breakthroughs only occurred during the past century and brings us to question what passed for medicines and curative procedures.

The European specie of leeches (from which Hirudotherapy gets its name) has long been used for medical purposes. Leech therapy dates back to the 1800s, where leech therapists typically used several leeches in each session. Leeches can consume as much as 10 to 15 ml of blood and expand dramatically in size. Once full, they automatically fall off the body, but can be removed using different methods. One technique used is applying salt or salt water, but this can make the leech vomit up the blood, which creates a higher risk of infection.

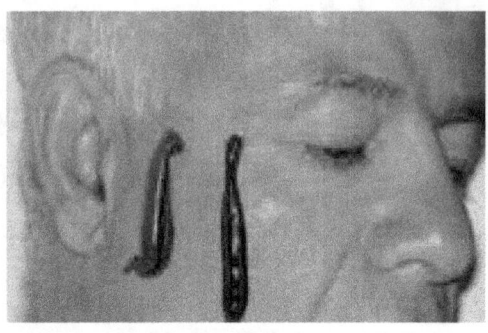

There are many benefits to Hirudotherapy, therefore making it extremely useful to treat various conditions. When a leech bites, its saliva is injected into the patient's bloodstream. This saliva contains Hirudin, which has an anticoagulant and hemodilution effect, preventing clot formation, which is very important because a clot can travel through the general circulation and block a blood vessel, thereby depriving organs of the necessary blood flow and the nutrients they need. This will cause ischemia and, eventually, failure of the organ involved. This can be fatal if the organ involved is the brain, heart or lungs as it can cause a stroke, heart attack or lung embolism.

Hirudin also helps reduce the blood's thickness, thereby promoting optimum blood flow and preventing the risks associated with sluggish blood flow.

LEECH THERAPY FOR PERIORBITAL HEMATOMA

One of the major features of leech therapy is the ability leeches have of extracting pooled blood. It also has an anti-edematous effect, which is especially helpful as a conservative measure to evacuate pooled blood as in the case of a periorbital hematoma.

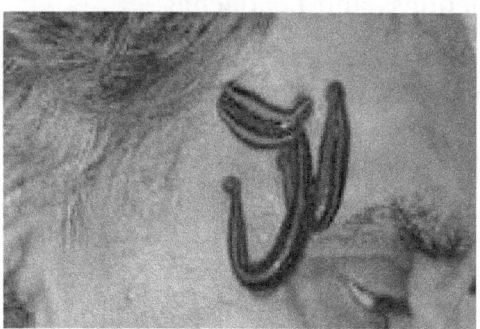

Periorbital hematoma is hematoma around the eyes - a sac of blood that the body creates to keep internal bleeding to a minimum. In most cases the sac of blood eventually dissolves, however, in some cases they may continue to grow or show no change. If the sac of blood does not disappear, then it may need to be surgically removed.

It usually occurs after a large amount of pressure or force has been applied to the area and something that is definitely common among boxers. This is shown by a bluish green discoloration around the eyes, more popularly known as the 'black eye.' Disappearance of pooled blood in this area is particularly slow and can take from several days to a few weeks. Not only is it unsightly, but can cause light-headedness and headaches.

Leech Therapy can be used to immediately evacuate the pooled blood around the eyes so the bluish-green discoloration can disappear after a mere couple of days.

PREVENT PROGRESS OF GLAUCOMA

Glaucoma is a condition that occurs when there is too much production of vitreous humor or when there's a very slow reabsorption of vitreous humor.

Vitreous humor is a transparent, jelly-like substance that gives nourishment to the eyes. Too much of it however, can be problematic, where the intra-ocular pressure can increase, causing compression of the eye structures. This causes gradual blurring of vision and slow but certain loss of sight.

Those at risk of developing glaucoma include diabetics, people over the age of 40, and people with a family history of the disease. If detected and treated in its early stages, glaucoma can be controlled and vision can be saved.

Leech Therapy can assist in the progression of this disease. The use of leeches to lessen the rate of blood flow to the eye lessens the production of vitreous humor and thus lessens the pressure inside the eye. Leech therapy can therefore help patients with glaucoma if this procedure is done in regular and frequent intervals and in conjunction with medicines that Ophthalmologists [medical eye specialists] prescribe to lessen the production of vitreous humor and lower the overall blood pressure in the area.

PREVENTING EYE INFLAMMATION

Another area where leech therapy can be beneficial is eye inflammation. Chorioretinitis [an inflammation of the choroid and retina of the eye], conjunctivitis [inflammation of the conjunctiva of one or both eyes], Keratitis [a condition in which the eye's cornea, the front part of the eye, becomes inflamed] and schleritis [a serious inflammatory disease that affects the white outer coating of the eye, known as the sclera] are just some of eye inflammation disorders.

Eye inflammations are inclined to have blood and other blood components pool in the affected area. This is the body's natural response, where it's attempting to fix whatever's wrong or damage in that area. Unfortunately, the pooling of too much blood causes significant change in the pressure inside the eye and this pressure causes compression and damage to other parts.

During Leech Therapy, blood is sucked out, thereby reducing inflammation. This leads to a reduction in pressure and lessens post-inflammatory complications.

Hirudotherapy also has a rejuvenating effect, where a feeling of vitality and renewed energy is felt by the patient. This is mainly due to relief from pain in certain treated conditions, as well as cleansing of the blood. There are no real explanations, but rather observations that over the centuries, Leech Therapy has indeed been used as a cure for many eye diseases.

LEECH THERAPY FOR SPORT INJURIES (GOFLER'S ELBOW)

Many athletes and sports enthusiasts experience injuries.

Injuries can occur due to body contact, poor co-ordination, trauma, lack of balance, repetitive movement, jolting or excessive force, but regardless, any kind of sport damage encounters pain to the injured part of the body, usually followed by inflammation and swelling.

Blood clots can also form as a response to tissue damage and when bleeding occurs, coagulation of blood takes place to block leakage, encouraging repair to damaged blood vessels.

Prolonged inflammation of an injured area can lead to a chronic condition and destruction of surrounding normal cells and tissues, further delaying the healing process, which can lead to a temporary loss of function.

Golfer's elbow is an inflammatory condition of the elbow caused by the same tendon being stressed during a game.

It can become very painful over time and unfortunately can interfere with a player's handicap, which is particularly frustrating for professional players as well as enthusiastic amateurs.

Usually, many players suffering golfer's elbow will try conservative treatment before resorting to anesthetics and steroids and in many cases will continue to feel pain due to the same tendon being continuously stressed during a golf swing.

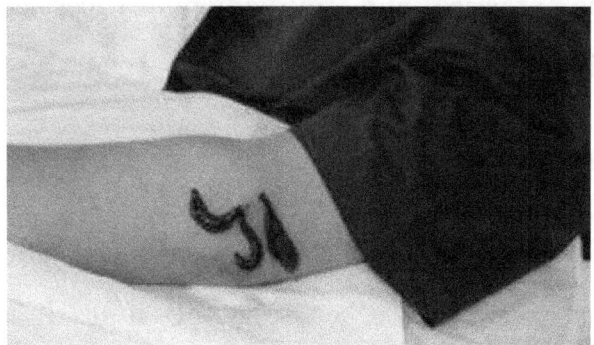

Leech Therapy is a safe and natural solution to Golfer's Elbow, without the need for continued visits to an occupational therapist or the use of anti-inflammatory drugs or steroids and most importantly, the requirement of resting the elbow for long periods, resulting in taking time away from the passion of the players.

Direct injuries caused by an external blow or force is very common in Rugby. Examples of collisions with other players during a tackle can cause haematomas [corks] and bruising, damage to joints and ligaments as well as dislocations and bone fractures.

During practice and tournaments, excessive and repetitive force can often be placed on the bones and other connective tissues of the body, causing overuse injury. In the early stages of these injuries, little or no pain might be experienced until the damage accumulates, causing the injured site to become inflamed and painful.

Leech therapy is extremely beneficial in the healing process of sport injuries due to enzymes found in leech saliva, which are known to reduce pain, inflammation and dissolving blood clots.

Enzymes found in leech saliva dilate vessels and work together with other enzymes to flush out toxins and promote healthy circulation to accelerate the healing process, as well as containing antibacterial enzymes that help prevent and eliminate the production of bacteria.

Leech therapy diminishes inflammation, swelling and pain of an injured area, leading to an accelerated normal function.

During therapy, leeches also inject an anesthetic enzyme which deadens the pain, as well as an antibacterial enzyme, which destroys the bacteria present, preventing further infection of the site, all of which work together to speed up the healing process of sport injuries.

Duration of leech therapy is dependent upon the severity of the sport injury. Likewise, the frequency of the sessions and the number of leeches used in the treatment also vary per individual.

LEECH THERAPY FOR MIGRAINE/ HEADACHES

Hirudotherapy excels in the treatment of migraine headaches. It is also quite useful with diseases of the peripheral nervous system in patients with acute stroke, with the trigeminal nerve, and polyneuropathy.

The leech creates a strong reflex action which acts as a muscle relaxant without causing damage to ligaments, tendons, or paraspinal muscles.

Hirudotherapy has a marked effect against swelling, which allows blood flow in previously affected areas. Leech saliva has a strong analgesic effect.

LEECH THERAPY FOR UROLOGICAL ISSUES

FOR MEN:

Many men experience an enlarged prostate which can lead to slow urination, decreased sexual drive, decreased fertility, and possibly prostate cancer down the road.

Adenoma (a benign tumor) and inflammation of the prostate gland usually result from venous stasis (slow blood flow) in the area.

Leeches are placed on the body, between the anus and the scrotum, and sometimes in the belly button and atop the liver/pancreas/spleen. The creatures' saliva injects a natural anti-inflammatory agent directly at the site to shrink the prostate. By restoring proper blood circulation in the area, leech therapy attacks the core of the disease.

How many sessions depends upon the condition. Nine sessions is typical. Non-severe cases are often treated once a week; severe cases are often treated every day or every other day.

FOR WOMEN:

Many women experience bladder infections. Leeches are applied between the anus and the vagina, and at the belly button and pubic bone. It is the antibiotic effect – without the side effects of drugs – that triggers the healing.

Seven to ten sessions is common; the effect is cumulative.

LEECH THERAPY IN GYNECOLOGY

Widespread use of synthetic hormones and antibiotic therapy, the problems of environmental toxins, and stress have led to the rapid spread of diseases and female genitalia.

These disorders often develop in conjunction with other chronic diseases, especially hypothyroidism, which complicates the course of these diseases.

Hirudotherapy has a powerful effect by reducing the load on the pelvic organs, preventing stagnation and inflammation. Hirudotherapy also has an immune-modulating effect.

Pain and discomfort in the abdomen, and genital itching generally disappear after the first session. After three or four months of treatment, we see a return to a normal menstrual cycle. We also see that pregnancy occurs in a previously infertile women.

There is a list of gynecological diseases for which hirudotherapy is helpful: chronic pelvic inflammatory disease, menstrual irregularities, adenomyosis (uterine thickening that occurs when endometrial tissue, which normally lines the uterus, moves into the outer muscular walls of the uterus), endometrial hyperplasia, functional ovarian cysts, uterine fibroids, some forms of infertility, menopausal syndrome, inflammatory diseases of the pelvic organs including viral and bacterial infections.

OTHER CONDITIONS SUITABLE FOR LEECH THERAPY

Respiratory system:

Acute and chronic bronchitis, bronchial asthma, pulmonary heart disease associated with chronic obstruction of the lungs and bronchial asthma, heavy pneumonia with difficulty breathing, Pickwickian syndrome, arteries with thrombosis (in the lungs), tuberculosis accompanied by blood vomiting.

Urinary system:

Pyelonephritis (type of urinary tract infection) with hypertension syndrome, hypostases (settling of the blood in relatively lower parts of an organ or body due to impaired circulation), chronic nephritic syndrome, cystitis (urinary bladder infection).

Musculoskeletal system:

Radiculitis (pain associated with nerves stemming out from the spine), arthritis.

Digestive system:

Hemorrhoids, pancreatitis, blood stasis in the liver, cirrhosis, cholecystitis (inflammation of the gallbladder), and other chronic inflammations of the abdominal cavity.

Cardiovascular system:

Asystole, Raynaud's disease, high blood pressure, stoppage of lymph flow, ischemic heart trouble, stenocardia, pre heart attack symptoms, heart attack, inflamed blood vessels, poor blood circulation, heart muscle diseases, obliterative arterial disease; obliterative thromboangitis, trophic ulcer of veins and arteries.

Obstetrics and gynecology:

Inflammatory conditions, complications during the postnatal period, problems with mammary glands, thrombophlebitis of the pelvic region, menopause. Also non-cancerous fibroids, endometriosis, adenomyosis, and ovarian cystic disease.

Dermatology:

Scleroderma, eczema, lupus, toxidermia, chronic dermatitis, psoriasis, erysipelatous inflammation of the skin.

Nose, Throat, Ears:

Acute and chronic pain of the auditory nerve, tinnitus, acute and chronic otitis, auditory canal infection, antritis, inflammation of the frontal sinuses, inflammation of cells in the ethmoid bone.

Ophthalmology:

Burst blood vessels in the eye, macular retinal dystrophy, inflammation of blood vessels in the eye, glaucoma.

Stomatology (diseases of the mouth):

Gingivitis, periodontitis, and acute and chronic cancer sores.

Surgery:

Postoperative blood clots, infiltration, and deficiency of blood flow after microsurgery and reconstructive surgery.

To fully understand why leech therapy works in such a wide range of applications, remember that the therapeutic activity of the leech is not based on a single mechanism of action, but on a combination of multiple effects. It reduces the viscosity of the blood while simultaneously dilating the blood vessels, accelerating lymph flow, inhibiting platelet aggregation, blocking numerous mediators of tissue infection, and exerting local analgesic and anesthetic effects, thus minimizing the pain of treatment. The medical term for such a cornucopia of effects is called a "multifactorial mechanism."

Allergies are the response to an immune system overreaction to an external substance. Allergies result in micro circulation and lymphatic malfunctions in the veins and venous system.

Bronchitis – both acute and chronic – are inflammatory conditions in the airways of the lungs, the bronchial tubes. Acute bronchitis is usually caused by viruses and certain bacteria. Chronic bronchitis is frequently a reaction to the environment and develops over time due to cigarette smoke, exposure to chemicals, and air pollution. Chronic bronchitis is most often an allergic reaction and it weakens the immune system, particularly in the elderly. When producing thick mucus, leech therapy can be very effective by strengthening the immune system, improving metabolism, and decreasing the venous plethora.

Gastritis is an inflammation of the stomach lining. It has many possible causes – unhealthy diet, accumulation of waste products in the body, and stress are common. It can lead to damage of the liver and gall bladder. A course of leech therapy may consist of 7 sessions.

Glaucoma is usually accompanied by a constant or periodic increase of intraocular pressure and nerve damage in the eye. The root cause is usually a poorly functioning regulation of fluid in the eye. Leech therapy acts a a defense against the primary causes of this disease by improving fluid circulation while reducing swelling.

Hemorrhoids are similar to varicose veins, but they affect the veins of the rectum. They are caused by high blood pressure in the veins of the anus. They can be internal or external. Typically a person with hemorrhoids has pain, swelling, inflammation, and bleeding. The person also may be prone to thrombosis and the buildup of blood clots. By placing leeches on the tailbone area, one is able to simultaneously drain the affected area and divert the blood flow, which in turn, has a strong healing effect. One patient who had undergone two surgeries and "tried everything" did not find relief until she began leech therapy.

Chronic pancreatitis is widespread. It affects the stomach's functions causing pain and an inability to properly digest and absorb food. Leech therapy has been shown to be an effective treatment, especially in the presence of blood stasis in the abdominal cavity.

Prostate enlargement is widespread. It is not uncommon to see an adenoma, a benign tumor. By restoring proper blood circulation to the area, leech therapy attacks the core of the disease.

Shingles (Herpes Zoster) requires timely treatment – within one week after the initial appearance of symptoms. A series of 4 to 5 treatments may be done at three- to four-day intervals.

Thrombophlebitis is caused by blood clots attacking a regular blood flow through the veins. There is hardly a better approach to this type of condition than the application of leech therapy. If leeches are applied in the early stages when only a reddening of the veins (phlebitis) is detected, then it is possible to prevent the development of blood clots.

Thrombosis – formation of a blood clot in a blood vessel – is a major cause of death and disability from heart attack (myocardial infarction), stroke, peripheral ischemia (narrowing of the arteries leading to lack of blood and oxygen getting to tissues), and pulmonary embolism (blockage of an artery in the lung). Standard heparin has been used successfully for the prevention and treatment of thrombotic disorders. However, its use has several limitations, including a variable anticoagulant effect, an inability to inhibit clot-bound thrombin, and the potential to cause thrombocytopenia. Direct thrombin inhibitors such as hirudin do not share these limitations.

Hirudin is the most potent non-covalent inhibitor of thrombin. It is a single peptide chain of 65 amino acids with molecular weight of ~7000. It is isolated from the salivary gland of the medicinal leech, Hirudo medicinalis. It selectively binds thrombin in a 1:1 fashion at each of two sites on the enzyme: 1) the domain that recognizes fibrinogen, and 2) the catalytic domain. Because of the specificity of binding, hirudin does not inhibit other enzymes in the coagulation or fibrinolytic pathways, such as factor Xa, factor IXa, kallikrein, activated protein C, plasmin or tissue-type plasminogen activator.

Tinnitus, or ringing of the ears, is said to be caused by different things, including exposure to loud noise, a build-up of ear wax, allergies, infection, trauma, high or low blood pressure, tumor, cardiovascular disease, or long-term use of certain medications such as aspirin and anti-inflammatories. Mechanically, it is thought to be a disruption of the tiny "hair" cells in the inner ear, or affecting the nerve pathways between the inner ear and the brain. Typically, leech therapy may consist of 6 sessions, a week or two apart.

Ulcers of the stomach and duodenum are often caused by weakening of the stomach wall. Leech therapy can be the primary treatment, especially when there are signs of inflammation. Or it can be a supplemental therapy used to accelerate the healing process.

Varicose veins are associated with a weakening of the structure of the veins' walls that cause them to stretch and swell. They are a sign that the entire circulatory system is stressed to some extent. Venous disease is one of the best-established traditional indications for leech therapy.

Wounds that are called non-healing are the results of circulatory problems and blood clots, and lead to the tissue's inability to health. Leeches improve micro circulation and blood circulation, while removing hypostasis, blood stasis, and stimulating the immune system which helps to clean and heal the wound.

THE MECHANICS OF LEECH THERAPY

The therapeutic effect of hirudotherapy is composed of several factors.

Hirudotherapy often makes use of the acupuncture points. Just as acupuncture uses a needle to bring more blood to the area, the action of the leeches likewise brings more blood to the area for healing. Leeches remove blood which prompts the liver to produce new, fresh blood.

When leeches bite, they create a tunnel to the lymphatic system remove toxins from the lymph system. This can be a profoundly effective means of systemic detoxification.

The creatures also deposit their saliva which contains a range of biologically active – healing – substances.

The leech's ability to sustain venous blood flow, in compromised skin flaps, is currently unmatched by any other means. The leech performs its service by physically evacuating blood and ensuring continued blood flow long after the leech detaches. The shape of the leech incision and substances in its saliva keep the blood flowing.

MECHANISM

Anticoagulants: Hirudin is one of many anti-clotting agents contained in the leech's saliva. Its purpose is to inhibit coagulation while the leech feeds. Hirudin has a high affinity for thrombin, binding and blocking its activity at very very low concentrations. Thrombin converts circulating fibrinogen into fibrin, creating an insoluble clot.

Other salivary components inhibit substances involved in platelet aggregation, including: adenosine diphosphate, epinephrine, platelet-activating factor and arachidonic acid.

Anesthetic: In the wild, leeches are usually not noticed by prey until they have been feeding for sometime. A natural anesthetic that minimizes host discomfort is presumed but as yet unidentified.

Anti-inflammatory: Leech saliva contains substances which inhibit the metabolism of arachidonic acid to prostaglandin. Prostaglandins are known to contribute to the pain, heat and swelling associated with the inflammatory process.

A number of small studies indicate that leech therapy may relieve the pain associated with osteoarthritis.

A leech can usually suck an average of 5 milliliters (ml) of blood within 15 to 60 minutes, but the real effect comes after the leech detaches. The bite can continue to bleed for up to 48 hours, releasing as much as 50 ml of blood. Usually treatments are carried out for 3 to 7 days, occasionally as long as 10 days. When the skin stays pink after leech therapy and venous oozing stops, the leech therapy can usually be discontinued.

The main effects of the medicinal leech on the body include:

❖ decreased blood clotting

- ❖ thrombolytic (clot destruction)
- ❖ antiischemic (improving blood supply to tissues and organs)
- ❖ antihypoxia (improved blood supply oxygen to the tissues and organs)
- ❖ hypertensive (normotensive)
- ❖ draining the blood and lymph system of toxins and blood clots
- ❖ restoration of the microcirculation
- ❖ recovery of neuromuscular impulse transmission
- ❖ restoration of vascular permeability
- ❖ bacteriostatic (death of microorganisms, causing inflammation)
- ❖ immunostimulatory

While the following isn't a complete list, the Hirudo Medicinalis is a small manufacturing factory of bioactive substances:

- ❖ Hirudin – Inhibits blood coagulant (binds to thrombin)

- ❖ Hyaluronidase – Lowers viscosity of hyaluronan (increasing tissue permeability); increases interstitial viscosity; antibiotic
- ❖ Apyrase – Inhibits host platelet aggregation
- ❖ Collagenase – Enzymes that break the peptide bonds in collagen
- ❖ Proteases – Enzymes for debridement of wounds and burns
- ❖ Lipolytic enzymes – Breakdown of lipids; involves the hydrolysis of triglycerides
- ❖ Destabilase – Dissolves fibrin (thrombolytic effects)
- ❖ Bdellines – Anti-inflammatory; inhibits trypsin, plasmin, acrosin
- ❖ Eglines – Anti-inflammatory; inhibit the activity of alpha-chymotrypsin, chymase, substilisin, elastase, cathepsin G
- ❖ Calin – inhibits blood coagulation (blocks the binding of van Willebrand factor to collagen). Inhibits collagen-mediated platelet aggregation

- ❖ Tryptase inhibitor – Inhibits proteolytic enzymes of host mast cells
- ❖ Factor Xa inhibitor — Inhibits the activity of coagulation factor Xa by forming equimolar complexes
- ❖ Acetylcholine – Vasodilator
- ❖ Carboxypeptidase A inhibitors – Increases the inflow of blood at the bite
- ❖ Leeches are pre-adapted to human physiology. The secretions from their saliva cross the entire spectrum of physiology: blood clotting, digestion, connective tissue, disease, pain, inhibition of enzymes, anti-inflammation.

There is a defined protocol for treating different diseases and conditions with leaches. The areas where the leaches are placed, the number of leeches used, and the number of sessions varies depending upon the condition being treated.

One leech will withdraw approximately one teaspoon of blood. For the next 12-48 hours, the site will discharge – it depends upon the person – up to about 16 tablespoons.

The application of a leech can take one minute, or twenty. Once the leech is attached, it will likely remain safely in place until fully distended. It will drop off usually within 30-60 minutes.

SAFETY CONCERNS REGARDING LEECH THERAPY

During a treatment session, one or more leeches are placed on the body in locations specific to the medical issue. Some patients report feeling a small pinch; others describe the feeling as similar to a mosquito bite. This is when the leech "hooks on."

Leeches will not hook on, by the way, if you have recently eaten garlic or if you have lotion or perfumes on your body so keep this mind when you come to your session.

There is a rhythmic pulling sensation as the leech begins feeding. In some cases the leech is removed in 2 minutes, in other cases, it may be left on for an hour and a half or until the leech naturally releases.

What the leech removes is approximately 30% blood and 70% toxins.

How deep do the leeches penetrate? They open your skin and go as deep as 1 1/2 milliliters.

The mark left behind looks like a three-pronged mark, something like the Mercedes automobile insignia. The mark fades away with time. We will wrap the treatment areas with a bandage.

Following treatment, there may be wound secretions. The fluid is typically blood, lymph, and a pus-like substance. It will very likely be dark in color. Most oozing occurs within 6 to 12 hours, however occasionally one might continue for up to 36 hours. It depends on the individual – the viscosity of your blood and how quiet you remain.

If you a more prolific discharger, then you may need to put a second bandage over the bandage we put on immediately after treatment. On the day of treatment, do not remove the first bandage, just apply a second. Stay quiet for the rest of the day and it is recommended that you do not go to work the following day.

Drink lots of water, or your choice of cranberry juice, blackcurrant juice, pomegranate juice, tomato juice, or coconut juice/water. Avoid alcohol. Please eat well and healthfully.

The day after treatment, you may take a shower and you can use 3% hydrogen peroxide (commonly sold in drug stores) to wipe and disinfect the area. Do not use rubbing alcohol. Cover the treatment area(s) with a small bandage in the event you continue to discharge.

You may experience slight swelling, itching, and superficial bruising. Itching is generally controlled with cold moist wraps or lemon juice – squeeze 1/2 of a lemon into 3 cups of water, dip a wash cloth in it and apply to the wound area. You can take Claritin or Benadryl (best in liquid form) if necessary for itching.

Do not touch the wound. Keep a bandage in place as long as there is oozing.

It is important to avoid scratching the area as it delays healing. Localized inflammation is relatively uncommon, however it can occur.

You might notice a temporary enlargement of the lymph nodes. This is part of the detoxification process and will go away on its own.

You might feel tired and sleepy, or energetic and vigorous. All of these reactions are common and normal.

Activities that cannot be performed on the day of a hirudotherapy session and for 48 hours after a session:

- ❖ physical therapy and/or massage, especially deep-tissue massage and/or lymphatic drainage
- ❖ reflexology
- ❖ aromatherapy, acupressure
- ❖ jogging
- ❖ biking
- ❖ intensive swimming
- ❖ weight-lifting
- ❖ running

After 2 days, resume normal activities unless you have been advised otherwise.

Case histories

1. The Vietnam veteran presented with high blood pressure on a 66 year old male even though his lifestyle was very disciplined: vegetarian eating, vegetable juicing, exercise, and lean body shape. When he took his B/P it was 150+/88. At the first session, the first B/P was 180/90 although he admitted to having "white coat syndrome." After the session (4 leeches) it was 139/80. On returning home, he periodically took readings, and the lowest (12 hours later) was 115/70. The second session (7 leeches) was seven days later. His B/P now stays near 130/80.

2. The woman presented with lymphatic stasis and varicosity in the lower extremities, with previous medical treatment of the small saphenous vein and surface varicosities. She had to wear medium compression stockings (knees down) due to pain and

swelling. Two days after the first session (6 leeches) her pain went from 10 to 3 without the need to wear stockings. After the second session (7 leeches) the pain dropped to .5 or 1 depending on work demands.

3. A clinical trial on patients with advanced osteoarthritis at the knee proved that leech therapy could effectively reduce the need for analgesic intake. It has been outlined that a double treatment regimen at a 4-week interval exhibited a longer term relieving and a better physical activity than a single treatment course. Moreover, the effectiveness of leech therapy in combination with the traditional Unani herbal formulation was also assessed. It was observed that patients who received the combined treatment displayed less pain and stiffness with better working ability. Other reports indicated leech therapy as an analgesic for iliosacral joints pain and cervicobrachialgia syndrome.

During an episode of food poisoning, the pain returned in her legs but resolved with another session. She has continued with treatments to detoxify the internal organs and reports feeling physically well and emotionally strong.

4. A recent case study showed how traditional Unani medicine, which includes leech therapy, was able to help save the foot of a 60-year-old woman with diabetes that faced amputation. Synthetic forms of leech saliva now exist, but researchers have discovered that using as few as four leeches in one session can help reduce the risk of amputation.

LEECH THERAPY: IS IT SAFE FOR YOU?

Present a random stranger with a leech and he'll most likely have disgust written all over his face. Tell him that you're going to let the leech bite him and he'll look at you as if you've given him a death threat. Indeed, people's reactions to leeches today are quite exaggerated and it's almost funny to see how people over react to this poor and simple creature with no backbone to speak of. All people would usually remember are blotched camping trips where skinny-dipping led to lots of screaming and thrashing around because their legs suddenly got decorated with little black bloodsuckers. But, really, leeches are relatively harmless - not only that, they're also very useful.

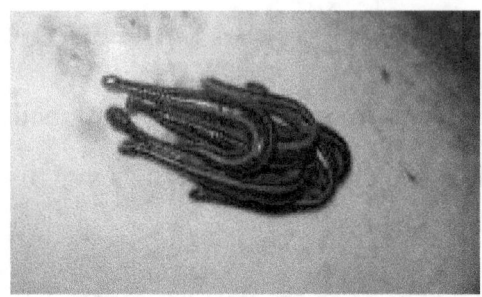

Leeches shown during treatment of
varied conditions

As you may have heard, the use of leeches in the field of medicine is widespread and very much accepted. They're popular in the field of plastic surgery, especially for cases where grafting is quite difficult and also for reconstructive surgery. They're also quite popular in microsurgery because of their ability to liquefy blood clots, thereby keeping the blood flowing and encouraging circulation.

But the idea of willingly letting a leech bite would be enough to make someone turn tail and run to the nearest exit. But really, leech therapy, aside from the minor inconveniences, is relatively harmless.

Pain

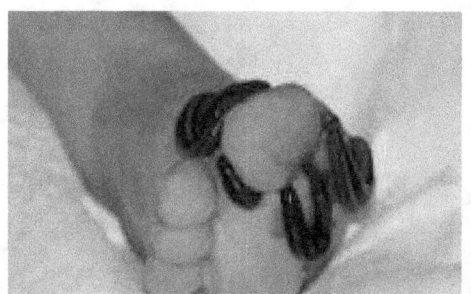

Leeches shown during treatment of
varied conditions

Of course, bites usually equate to pain and a leech's bite is no exception, however, the pain that stems from a leech's bite is slight. Some people say that it's hardly noticeable and others say that it hurts as much as a wasp's sting - but this is rather rare. The slight stinging sensation of a leech's bite usually lasts for only about one to five minutes and after that, their natural local anesthetic effect kicks in. Usually, a patient's pain is connected to their anxiety before the procedure, so simply put, the more you dread it, the more it hurts! So, the best thing is to try and distract yourself whenever leeches are applied and you probably won't feel a thing.

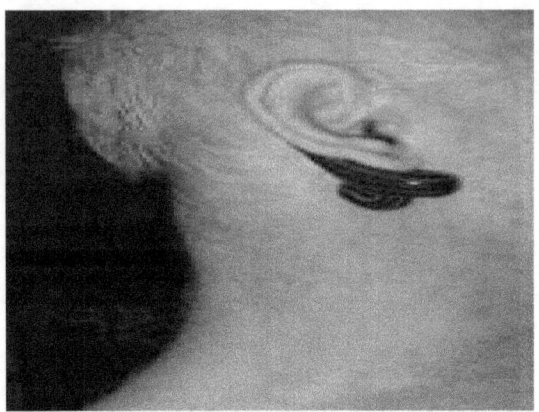

Leeches shown during treatment
of varied conditions

Pruritus [Itchiness]

Itching on the site of the bite for the first few days
is a common side effect of leech therapy. It's not an
allergic reaction, though people often mistake it to
be so and it's advised that the patient should be
advised to avoid scratching the area because it delays
wound healing. Local natural remedies for itching
can be used, like cold moist wraps or vinegar wraps
and if the itching is intense, antipruritic drugs like
Fenistil ointment or an oral antihistamine can be
used.

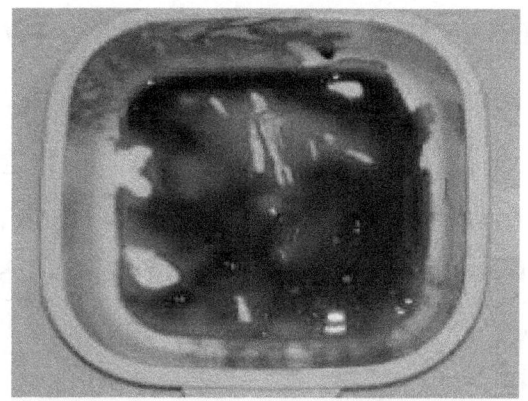

Blood expelled after different treatments

Blood Loss

Leeches are blood suckers, meaning that whenever they attach to your skin, they ingest some of your blood. Now, in the wild imaginations of people who abhor creepy crawly things, leeches can suck a person's blood until the person shrivels up and dies, but of course, we know that this is really not the case! Leeches only suck about a teaspoon of blood and when they're full, they naturally fall off. Of course leeches also have an enzyme called Hirudin in their saliva, which is an anticoagulant that is injected into a person's bloodstream. However, blood may keep seeping several hours after the bite, which may cause some anxiety for the patient, but is nothing to worry about.

THE BENEFITS OF LEECH THERAPY AND ITS EFFECTS

Yes, leeches can be thought of as slimy and unattractive creatures, but ugly or not, they do serve a lot of medical purposes when it comes to us, humans.

Since ancient times, leeches were used to treat many illnesses and disease through bloodletting, a method where blood was drawn out in the hope that removing impure blood would heal the body. Believe it or not, leech therapy is sometimes the best alternative in treating illnesses, and even surpasses pharmacological treatments. Because of its healing effects to the human body, this traditional method of curing diseases is still thriving today.

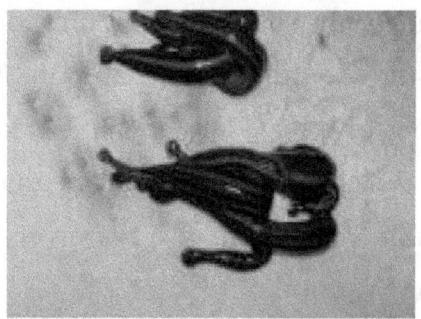

Leeches shown during treatment

THE BENEFITS

There are more than 600 species of leeches that have been identified, but only 15 of the species are used medically, so they are given a class of their own. They are classified as Hirudo Medicinalis or medicinal leeches.

Leech therapy has been used and is still in use for many diseases of the body. They are used to treat arthritis and other inflammatory processes. It is perfect for those with vascular (arterial and venous diseases), heart (ischemic diseases and hypertension). The GI or gastrointestinal tract can also benefit from leech therapy, especially those who suffer from hepatitis, stomach ulcers, and pancreatitis, among others. Likewise, individuals with problems in their genitourinary system and gynecological disorders will also benefit greatly from leech therapy. Skin diseases like psoriasis, herpes, and eczema can also be treated with leech therapy. Other problems known to benefit from leech therapy are the eyes (example is glaucoma) and the brain (for infantile cerebral palsy).

But how exactly do leeches treat these many illnesses and diseases?

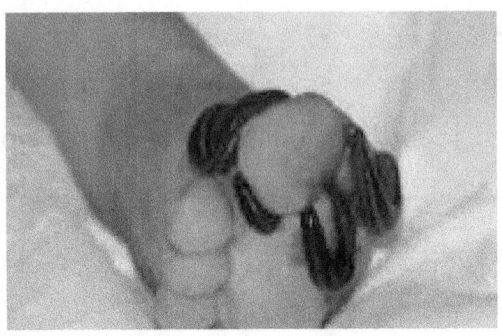

Leeches shown during treatment of
varied conditions

Anticoagulating Effects of Leeches

The leech's saliva contains enzymes and compounds
that act as an anticoagulation agent. The most
prominent of these anticoagulation agents is hirudin,
which binds itself to thrombins, thus, effectively
inhibiting coagulation of the blood.

Another compound that prevents coagulation is
calin. This, on the other hand, works as an
anticoagulant by prohibiting the von Willebrand
factor to bind itself to collagen, and it is also an
effective inhibitor of platelet aggregation caused by
collagen.

The saliva of the leeches also contains Factor Xa inhibitor which also blocks the action of the coagulation factor Xa.

Clot Dissolving Effects of Leeches

The action of destabilase is to break up any fibrins that have formed. It also has a thrombolytic effect, which can also dissolve clots of blood that have formed.

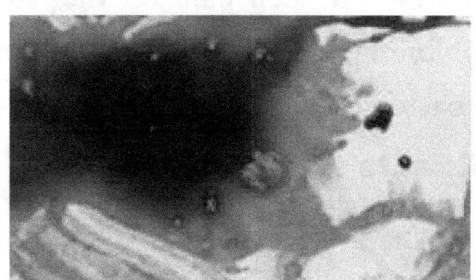

Blood expelled after different treatments

Anti-inflammatory Effects of Leeches

Bdellins is a compound in the leech's saliva that acts as an anti-inflammatory agent by inhibiting trypsin as well as plasmin. It also inhibits the action of the acrosin. Another anti-inflammatory agent is the eglins.

Vasodilating Effects of Leeches

There are three compounds in the leeches' saliva that act as a vasodilator agent, and they are the histamine-like substances, the acetylcholine, and the carboxypeptidase A inhibitors. All these act to widen the vessels, thus, causing inflow of blood to the site.

Bacteriostatic and Anesthetic Effects of Leeches

The saliva of leeches also contains anesthetic substances which deaden pain on the site and also bacteria-inhibiting substances which inhibit the growth of bacteria.

Overall Effects to the Human Body

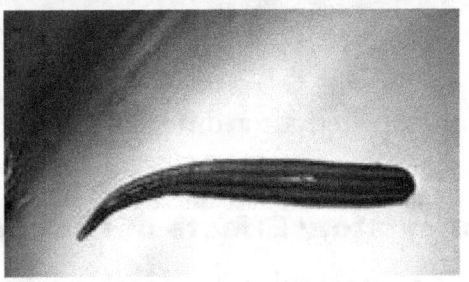

Medicinal leech grown to 13cm
after treatment

Once the leeches attach themselves to the skin of the patient and start sucking blood, the saliva enters the puncture site and along with it the enzymes and compounds responsible for all these positive effects. Working together, they act to cure the disease present in the individual. Because of anticoagulation agents, the blood becomes thinner, allowing it to flow freely through the vessels. The anti-clotting agents also dissolve clots found in the vessels, eliminating the risk of them traveling to other parts of the body and blocking an artery or vein. The vasodilating agents help widen the vessel walls by dilating them, and this causes the blood to flow unimpeded, too.

Patients who suffer from pain and inflammation will feel relief from the anti-inflammatory and anesthetic effects of the leech's saliva.

In the long run, leech therapy also helps to normalize the blood pressure of hypertensive individuals as well as lessen their risk of suffering from stroke and heart attacks. Blood circulation is also improved with leech therapy and it helps with the healing process of wounds, as well as wounds and lesions caused by diabetes. There is also a noticeable boost in the immune system's function due to bacteriostatic agents.

Infection

A leech's body contains bacteria that may cause infection, but these microorganisms are easily killed by antibiotics, therefore it's quite safe to use leech therapy.

STANDARD OPERATIVE PROCEDURE (SOPs)

Accelerating use and acceptance of leech therapy in mass needs rational presentation, aseptic procedures and safety assurance. So development of standard operative procedure regarding the leech therapy is need of hour. Decision to advice Leech therapy for a selective disease, selection of medicinal leeches, number of leeches, site of applications, duration for which leeches should be used and the whole procedure of leech application till the removal of leech comes under SOPs. Two heading can be framed for leeching procedure.

I.Selection of Leeches

II.Procedure of Leeching

I. SELECTION OF LEECHES

Types of leeches: The leeches are hermaphrodite as earth worm (have both male and female elements). As per *Unani* medicine two types of leeches are found one those are therapeutically usable called as "medicinal leeches" and rest is non-medicinal or poisonous leeches. Medicinal leeches are needed to separate from non medicinal leeches. *Hirudo medicinalis* and *Hirudinaria granulosa* species are commonly known medicinal leeches; these medical leeches are haemophagic parasitic "blood sucking" and have been used in *Unani* system of medicine since centuries. The medicinal leeches found in fresh water, leech saliva contains anticoagulant, vasodilators, lipotropic and anaesthetic properties. Medicinal leeches have two suckers, one at each end. The caudal (Back end) end has suction cup which helps the leeches to ambulate (crawling) and to attach to its host. The frontal end which also known as rostral suction cup also contains the mouth with three sharp jaws that leaved a 'Y' shaped mark.

Features of therapeutically usable leeches

- According to *Unani* physicians the leeches should have following feature for medicinal purposes

- The leeches should be trapped from the clean water where algae / moss are abundantly present

- The pond should also have frogs

- The colour of leeches should be *Masheeul laun* (colored like seed of *Vigna radiata*), greenish and with two golden colored strip on the body.

- We can select those leeches also which are of hepatic colored.

- We can select those leeches also which are like a Rat's tail in its fineness and roundness.

- Leeches should be thin and small headed

- With emerald green and rounded side.

PROCEDURE OF LEECH THERAPY

It can be divided as follows;

1. Pre-leeching procedure

2. Leeching procedure

3. Post-leeching procedure

1. Pre leeching procedure:

Ideally aseptic and separate room should be there which is well equipped with

- Patient bed

- Separate tank/bottles for leech storage

- The dressing trolley which is having sterilized gloves, sterilized gauze pieces, normal saline, turmeric powder, *sufoof habisuddam*, dressing material, BP instrument, emergency medicines etc.

- Doctor should wear the sterilized apron.

- Examination & Investigations

- Examine vitals and blood pressure

- Important investigations which should be done before leeching process (last three are optional).

- Hemoglobin estimation to avoid anemic patients. Hb % should be done on every 15th day during treatment.

- BT, CT, BS level. To detect and avoid patients having diabetes, hemophilia and other diseases.

- HIV test to avoid cross infection

- Complete haemogram

- HBsAg avoid cross infection

Preparation of leeches: According to *Unani* literature leeches should be collected just one day before the use

- The collected leeches dropped in a wide mouth kidney like tray or bowel filled with clean water.

- Use palatable water which is free from contaminations and chlorination because it can kill the leech. Water should be changed every 3rd day.

- Fine turmeric powder is mixed in it. One can observe that an inactive leech become active and runs all around the tray immediately after sprinkling of the powder which indicates its carving for food.

- After this, the active leeches are selected and transferred in another tray having clean water.

- Preparation of the patient

- Selection of suitable patient

- Light semi solid diet before the procedure should be advised.

- Disorders like anemia, hemophilia, Diabetes Mellitus, Hepatitis and HIV etc. should be ruled out by appropriate investigations.

- The desired site should be washed with cold water properly.

- Spirit gauze or turmeric should not be used for cleaning the application site.

2. Leeching procedures

- Take towel, soap, gauze pieces, powder of natural anticoagulant (like *Geru* (red Chalk), *Murdarsang* and Alum) and sterile needle.

- The desired site is cleaned with wet gauze.

- Now, the leech is held at its neck with fingers and applied directly to the skin.

- Once leeches start sucking the blood, they are covered with wet gauze and cold water is poured on them from above time to time, so as to make leech comfortable during sucking.

- If leech do not catch the site by its own, then rub the site of leeching to increase blood circulation of that particular area or a small prick induced bleeding may be required so as to facilitate the sucking procedure.

- The leech when once starts sucking the blood, elevates its neck, and fixes its head to the supporting point of skin. One can observe wave like movements indicating sucking of blood.

- Leave it for 30 minutes to 60 minutes.

- When leech become fully satisfied with its food, it leaves off the skin of the patient and drops itself down.

- If this not happen, then the patient may feel itching sensation which indicates impure blood from that spot is no more available for the leech.

- In such a case, a little turmeric powder is sprinkled on the sucking point of the leech and immediately the leech takes away its mouth from that point.

3. Post leeching procedure

For patients

- Leech is removed from the site

- The site is cleaned with normal saline or other antiseptic solution.

- Turmeric powder is sprinkled to the bleeding site

- Bandaging is done to arrest the bleeding (some physicians suggest that blood is allowed for some time to ooze after removal of leech)

- Sips of lime water, soup, or glucose water can be offered to the patient

- Patient is allowed to sit for few minutes before leaving the place.

For leeches (Post procedure leech care)

- Leeches after use are kept in an empty tray.

- Turmeric powder is sprinkled on its mouth just to induce vomiting so that it vomits the blood.

- Some of the practitioners advocate to gently squeezing out the blood with fingers from anus to mouth.

- After this the leech is again washed in clean water.

- At the end leech is transferred in the separate jar and kept starving for normally seven days.

- Please keep the leeches in separate container of each patient with their name tag or code and date of starting the procedure.

COMPLICATIONS

Although leech therapy is an innovative and safe approach in medical science and promising for various ailments but its use is accompanied by various complications too. The most common may be:

- Prolonged bleeding.

- Allergic reactions and bacterial infections. The bacteria aeromonas-hydrophilia present in gut of leech can cause pneumonia, septicemia or gastroenteritis.

- Allergic reactions such as itching followed by burning and blister formation and ulcerative necrosis due to toxins present in leech saliva have also been reported after leech therapy.

- Transmission of certain infections from one subject to the other is another probable complication of leech therapy. Hence, it is mandatory to rule out the selected cases for certain conditions by performing a series of required hematological or serological investigations.

- Few such conditions include various blood borne infections like HIV and Hepatitis, blood disorders like hemophilia, thrombocytopenia and conditions like pregnancy and anemia.

But if we follow the standard operative procedure; chances of complications and side effects are almost negligible.

CONTRAINDICATIONS FOR LEECH THERAPY

- ❖ Hemophilia
- ❖ Leukemia

- ❖ Multiple Myeloma
- ❖ Lymphoma
- ❖ Low blood pressure
- ❖ Anemia
- ❖ HIV-infection-AIDS
- ❖ Chemotherapy
- ❖ Liver Cancer
- ❖ Pacemaker
- ❖ Pregnancy
- ❖ Menstrual period

Do not apply leeches if client is on the following medication:

- ❖ Coumadin
- ❖ Plavix
- ❖ Lovenox
- ❖ Marcumar or similar are in use

The Hirudin enzyme in leech salivary gland secretion works similarly to Heparin and is 10 times more powerful than commonly used anticoagulants. Consequently, the two blood thinners cannot be applied at the same time. You do not need a physician's consent to stop intake of aspirin, Viagra, fish oil, and ginkgo biloba.

If gingko biloba products, aspirin, fish oil, Viagra are in use, you should stop taking them 2-3 days before the leech therapy begins.

Please inform to your physician if you take any of the following:

- ❖ Anti-inflammatory and antidepressant medication
- ❖ Strong pain-reliever drugs
- ❖ Chinese, Unani herbs
- ❖ Alternative healing creams
- ❖ Homeopathic remedies

Some detoxification diets must not be in progress during hirudotherapy. Notify your physician if you are on any special diet including the following:

- ❖ Starvation diet
- ❖ Juices-only diet

- ❖ Cleansing diet
- ❖ Dietary supplements diet
- ❖ Colon hydrotherapy
- ❖ Cortisone therapy
- ❖ Prednisone therapy (for migraine headache)
- ❖ Liver cleansing
- ❖ Kidney cleansing and/or any other detox
- ❖ Lymphatic drainage
- ❖ Chelation therapy
- ❖ Acupuncture
- ❖ Bee venom therapy
- ❖ Tranquilizers & steroids therapy

The following activities cannot be done on the day of or for two days after a leech session:

- ❖ Physical therapy
- ❖ Intense massage
- ❖ Deep-tissue massage
- ❖ Reflexo-therapy
- ❖ Aromatherapy
- ❖ Acupressure

- ❖ Jogging
- ❖ Biking
- ❖ Intensive swimming
- ❖ Weight-lifting
- ❖ Intensive running

Also notify your physician of any medical issues, including the use of a pacemaker and having very low blood pressure.

CONCLUSION

To conclude, leeching is a popular therapeutic practice throughout the ages for a wide range for diseases and it can be applied as an unscientific home remedy by traditional therapists. Nowadays, leech came back to the contemporary medicine with fewer applications, which were proven and supported by a huge number of scientific studies and case reports. Leech therapy in the field of plastic and reconstructive surgery is expected to be of paramount importance due to the ease of leech application and reduced side-effects. Hence, more efforts should be undertaken to optimize this utilization. More investigations are required also to assess leech efficacy and safety in the management of diseases.

Nowadays, leeches are used successfully for only a few conditions, notably in the field of reconstructive or microsurgery, to salvage tissue flaps and skin grafts whose viability is threatened by venous congestion. The anticoagulant properties of hirudin, contained in leech saliva, may lead to wider therapeutic applications in the prevention and treatment of thromboembolic diseases. However, its application in dentistry is yet unexplored and this should motivate further research on its use in treatment of various dental disorders. At the same time optimal care should be taken when applying leeches, because their use can be associated with serious complications.

REFERENCES

1. Andereya S, Stanzel S, Maus U, Mueller-Rath R, Mumme T, Siebert CH, et al. Assessment of leech therapy for knee osteoarthritis: A randomized study. Acta Orthop. 2008;79:235–43.

2. Zaidi S, Jamil S, Sultana A, Zaman F, Fuzail M. Safety and efficacy of leeching therapy for symptomatic knee osteoarthritis using Indian medicinal leech. Indian J Tradit Knowledge. 2009;8:437–42.

3. http://arizonaleechtherapy.com

4. Yule CM, Yong HS. Kaula Lampur: Akademi Sains Malaysia; 2004. Freshwater Invertebrates of the Malaysian Region.

5. Sawyer RT. Leech Biology and Behaviour. Vol. 2. Michigan: Clarendon Press; 1986. Feeding, biology, ecology and systematics.

6. Rouse G, Pleijel F. Enfield, USA: Science Publishers; 2006. Reproductive Biology and Phylogeny of Annelida.

7. Britanica. Leech: Encyclopedia Britanica. 2012. [Cited on 2012 Mar 31]. Available from: http://www.britannica.com/EBchecked/topic/334632/leech .

8. http://www.ncbi.nlm.nih.gov/pmc/articles

9. Tanzeel A, Anwar M. Clinical Importance of Leech Therapy. IJTK 2009; 8(3):443-445.

10. Ibn Sina. Al Qanoon fil Tib. (Urdu translation. by Kantoori GH). Vol. II; New Delhi: Aijaz publishing house; 2007:2-10,47.

11. Lone AH. Ahmad T, Anwar M, Habib S. Sofi G, Imam H. Leech Therapy- A Holistic Approach of Treatment in Unani (Greeko-Arab) Medicine. Ancient Science of Life, 2013; 31(1): 31-35.

12. Magner LN. History of Medicine. New York. Marcel Dekker. 1992:4, 203-5.

13. Zarnigar, Anwar MA. Effect of Taleeq (Leech Therapy) in Dawali (Varicose Veins). Ancient Science of Life; 30(3): 84-91.

14. Md Tanwir Alam, Hasan I, Perveen Aisha, Nazamudduin and Perveen Shaista. Leech Therapy (Taleeq): Indication, Contraindication and Standard Operative Procedures (SOPs).

www.ingramcontent.com/pod-product-compliance
Lightning Source LLC
Chambersburg PA
CBHW070808180526
45168CB00002B/534